Co

CW00326586

What is psoriasis?

Being told you have the skin condition psoriasis can be devastating. We all tend to have an image of psoriasis based on very severe cases such as the playwright Dennis Potter, who died in 1994. But, although it inevitably takes some time to adjust to the diagnosis, you can take some comfort from knowing that psoriasis usually comes and goes, occasionally disappears forever, and varies from very mild to the much rarer, more severe forms.

Psoriasis is surprisingly common, affecting one to three per cent of most populations in the world. It tends to be particularly common in Europe and the USA and least common in black West Africans and Latin Americans. Psoriasis affects men and women equally. It can start at any age, but often occurs for the first time in five- to nine-year-old girls and in 15- to 19-year-old boys. It can

also start for the first time in men and women between the ages of 57 and 60 years.

No one knows for certain what causes psoriasis. You can inherit the tendency to have the condition, so psoriasis may run in your family. This tendency is then activated by an infection, certain drugs or stress, although it is often impossible to identify specific triggers. There are also some abnormalities of chemicals in skin cells that interact and contribute to the characteristic skin changes seen in psoriasis. One thing is for certain, there is no virus or bacterium involved. You cannot catch psoriasis from others, and you cannot infect others with psoriasis if you have the condition yourself.

Psoriasis causes pink or red, raised patches of skin. These patches look very distinct from the rest of the normal-looking skin because they have a well-defined edge around them. They are called 'plaques' by doctors. The plaques have a scaly surface and may range in size from tiny to very large. Some people with psoriasis also experience itching.

The plaques are caused by abnormal skin cell replacement. Your skin constantly replaces its outermost layer (the epidermis) because the cells get rubbed off while you go about your daily life. In people with psoriasis, the epidermal cells are replaced too quickly and over-enthusiastically. The cells that come to the surface are not properly formed and get heaped up into the plaques. Underlying blood vessels are also damaged, causing the redness that often occurs in psoriasis. White blood cells, which move into the the plaques, can form clear blisters or pustules in the epidermis. These blisters or pustules may appear on the soles of the feet and palms of the hands. These same changes can also occur in the nails, which may become thickened and damaged, and contain tiny pits. A minority of people with psoriasis also develop joint problems – for more on this, see 'Psoriasis and other diseases + lifestyle issues' on page 46.

It is very hard to predict whether your psoriasis will worsen, improve or stay the same throughout your life. Psoriasis tends to remain a long-standing (chronic) problem, although there are usually some periods when it is much better and others when it flares up.

There is no overall cure for psoriasis, although it does sometimes just disappear of its own accord. However, the treatments have greatly improved in recent years, and although coping with psoriasis is still a great challenge for many, the help available is better now than it has ever been before.

KEY POINTS

✓ Psoriasis affects one to three per cent of the population

✓ It produces red and scaly patches

✓ It is not infectious

Skin changes in psoriasis

NORMAL SKIN

The skin is your largest organ, weighing about four kilograms and covering about two square metres. It is your interface with the environment, protecting you against chemicals, bacteria and radiation, helping you to maintain a stable body temperature, and stopping you from losing fluid and vital body chemicals. Your skin contains nerve endings that allow you to feel objects. Nails, which are also part of your skin layer, enable you to prise things open.

The skin is waterproof, strong and resilient, yet also flexible. It consists of two layers of cells. The

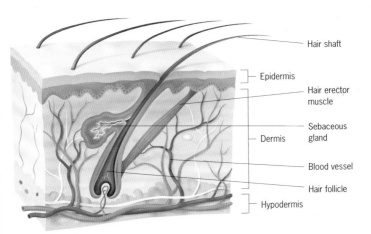

Hair shaft

Epidermis

Hair erector muscle

Sebaceous gland

Dermis

Blood vessel

Hair follicle

Hypodermis

Your skin protects you against chemicals, bacteria and radiation, helps you maintain a stable body temperature, and stops you from losing fluid and vital body chemicals.

outer layer is called the epidermis and is made up of epithelial cells. The epidermis is supported from below by the dermis, which is a network of elastic fibres, blood vessels, hair follicles and roots, nerve endings, and sweat and lymph glands. Underneath the dermis, there is another layer of cells known as the hypodermis, which contains loose connective tissue and fat.

The epidermis contains many layers of closely packed cells. The cells nearest the skin's surface are flat and filled with a hard substance called keratin. The epidermis contains no blood vessels – these are all in the dermis and deeper layers. The epidermis is thick in some parts (one millimetre thick on the palms and soles) and thin in others (just 0.1 millimetre thick over the eyelids). Dead cells are shed from the surface of the epidermis as very fine scale, and are replaced by other cells that pass from the deepest (basal) layers to the surface layers over a period of four weeks.

SKIN CHANGES

What is going on in the skin of people with psoriasis to produce the red scaly plaques? The epidermis in psoriatic skin is turning over much more rapidly compared with normal skin – possibly seven times as fast. This results in the epidermal cells not having time to mature fully. Instead of normal virtually invisible scale being formed, in people with psoriasis the resulting scale is visible, white and loose,

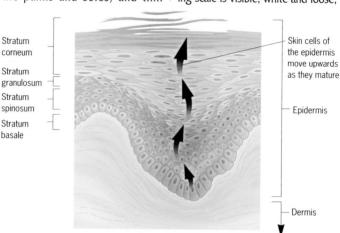

Stratum corneum

Stratum granulosum

Stratum spinosum

Stratum basale

Skin cells of the epidermis move upwards as they mature

Epidermis

Dermis

Dead cells are shed from the surface of the epidermis as a fine scale and are replaced by other cells that pass from the deepest layers to the surface layers over a period of about four weeks.

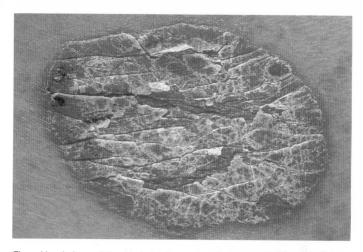

The epidermis in psoriatic skin is turning over much more rapidly than normal skin. Immature skin cells reach the surface forming plaques of loose visible scale.

and can be removed easily by gently scraping over the plaques.

Plaques look silvery and scaly because they are full of immature skin cells. If some skin cells are removed from a plaque of psoriasis (a technique called a biopsy), there are signs of increased cell turnover and inflammation. The increased cell turnover is shown by an increase in the dividing cells that form keratin (keratinocytes). There are also signs that the epidermal cells do not mature fully. Their immaturity is characterised by the presence of their nuclei, which contain the cells' genetic material. As skin cells travel from the basal layers to the epidermis, their nuclei usually disappear. The outer layers of the plaques still have nuclei present, known as

parakeratosis, and this shows that the cells have made their way up to the skin's surface too quickly; this gives rise to the silvery scale already described.

Plaques may also look red because, in psoriasis, the blood vessels in the dermis are dilated (enlarged). This causes an increased blood flow, which gives the plaques their red colour.

INFLAMMATORY CHANGES

There is considerable inflammation in psoriasis. This causes the red, irritated plaques. No one is quite certain whether the abnormal skin in psoriasis is caused by a dysfunction of the immune system (an oversensitivity reaction, for example) or whether the immune system is activated because the skin is abnormal.

Either way, many cells that usually fight infections and repair injuries to the skin are found in the epidermis of people with psoriasis.

White blood cells called T lymphocytes (T cells) are often found in the dermis of affected people. The drug cyclosporin A, which can be very beneficial in severe psoriasis, counteracts these T cells. This suggests that the cells may be playing a role in the development of psoriasis.

As mentioned, increased cell turnover is the main cause of the red and scaly plaques of psoriasis. However, clinical studies and skin biopsies suggest that immunological changes may also be involved. Therefore, many of the treatments of psoriasis are directed against the increased cell turnover, the immunological factors or a mixture of the two.

KEY POINTS

✓ In psoriasis, the skin renews itself in four days instead of 28 days

✓ The silvery, scaly patches of skin are called plaques

✓ Plaques consist of immature skin cells

✓ Inflammation may play a role in the formation of plaques

What causes psoriasis?

No one really knows for certain what causes psoriasis. But there are two factors that may contribute to the development of the condition, namely (1) genetic predisposition and (2) triggers that make psoriasis appear.

GENETIC PREDISPOSITION

Psoriasis often, but not always, runs in families. However, the inheritance of psoriasis is not predictable because the abnormalities that cause it are carried on several different genes. There is no single gene that can be tested to predict with certainty whether you'll get psoriasis or not. If you have several members of your family who have psoriasis, you are more likely to have psoriasis than someone who has no affected relatives – but it is by no means certain that you'll ever get it.

Similarly, some people develop psoriasis out of the blue, and have no other relatives they can think of who've ever had the condition. In fact, only around one-third of people with psoriasis can think of any family members with the condition. In this sense, the inheritance of psoriasis is like that of eye colour. If you have two parents with brown eyes, you and your siblings are likely to have brown eyes too, but this is not definitely the case. You may have hazel or blue eyes because – as with psoriasis – eye colour is carried on several genes and has an unpredictable pattern of inheritance. However, the fact that genetics is involved means that psoriasis is more likely to develop in individuals who have many affected close family members.

The most powerful genetic evidence arises from twin studies. If a non-identical twin has psoriasis, then the other twin has a 20 per cent chance of developing psoriasis. If the twins are identical, however, the risk rises to 73 per cent. Non-identical twins are genetically similar to ordinary brothers and sisters, whereas identical twins are identical because they literally have the same genes. Perhaps it is surprising that in identical twins it is only a 73 per cent and not a 100 per cent risk – this indicates that there are other, probably environmental, factors involved.

It seems that what happens is that you inherit a tendency to psoriasis. The condition develops only if you are exposed to specific triggers in the environment, such as viral illnesses, certain drugs or stress.

If your child has psoriasis, you may want to know whether any other children in your family are likely to develop the condition too. If a child has developed psoriasis, and if both parents have psoriasis, the chances of another sibling developing the condition is 50 per cent (the incidence of psoriasis in the general population is only about two per cent). If, however, only one parent has psoriasis, the chances of a sibling developing the condition is 16.4 per cent. If a child with psoriasis has no parents with psoriasis, then the risk of the sibling being affected falls to 7.8 per cent.

If you have a sibling who has psoriasis, you will be wondering how likely you are to develop psoriasis yourself. The answer depends on what age your sibling developed the condition for the first time. If your brother or sister first developed psoriasis before they were 15, your risk of developing it yourself is three times higher than if your brother or sister developed it for the first time when they were over 30.

Recent molecular genetic studies have shown that the tendency to have psoriasis is linked to certain genes found at sites on the long arms of two specific chromosomes (thread-like structures carrying several genes): chromosome 17 and chromosome 4. However, this has applied only in families where there are a large number of members with psoriasis. These findings have not been confirmed in the general population. Therefore, a genetic test for the condition is still a long way off.

TRIGGERS THAT CAUSE PSORIASIS

If you have a genetic predisposition to develop psoriasis, certain triggers may activate the condition. However, in the vast majority of people who develop psoriasis, the relevant triggers cannot be identified.

Streptococcal infection

Streptococcal infection, which is a common cause of sore throats and tonsillitis, is a clear trigger in some people, particularly in children and young adults. The type of psoriasis that is most typically induced is guttate psoriasis, the rash appearing about ten days after the streptococcal tonsillitis. In patients with the more common plaque psoriasis, it is rare for streptococcal infection to be the trigger.

Hormonal factors
There is a peak onset of psoriasis at the menarche (when the periods start) and the menopause (when the periods stop). Psoriasis tends to improve in pregnancy and worsen after delivery. However, this is by no means invariable and there are no clear-cut hormonal triggers.

'Trauma' to the skin
If the skin is injured, psoriasis may develop. This is known as the Köbner reaction – for more details, see page 21.

Sun exposure
Ultraviolet light helps the vast majority of people with psoriasis. However, a few people (less than five per cent) notice that even small amounts of sunlight – at levels that do not cause sunburn – aggravate their condition. Some people will have psoriasis only on areas of their skin that are often exposed to the sun, such as their face, hands and forearms. If a person is sunburnt, there is a risk that the psoriasis will flare up because of the Köbner reaction.

Drugs
Some drugs worsen already existing psoriasis. This applies particularly to lithium, which is commonly used in the management of people with manic depression. If you have been taking corticosteroid drugs by mouth for other conditions, you may find that your psoriasis flares up when the corticosteroids are withdrawn. The same reaction may occur if you have been using potent topical steroid creams and ointments on your skin – if you suddenly stop using topical steroids, a nasty and often pustular flare-up of your psoriasis can result.

Psychological factors
It is always difficult to prove a relationship of the mind to psoriasis, and indeed to most skin disorders. Undoubtedly, in some people, psychological factors are important and they notice that when they are under stress their psoriasis worsens. On the other hand, it is stressful to have an unpleasant skin disease, so it is hard to sort out the cause and effect. In individual patients, stress can be a clear aggravating factor, but, for the majority, it is not a strong trigger of psoriasis.

✓ There are strong genetic factors

✓ Psoriasis can be triggered by streptococcal tonsillitis

✓ Lithium treatment of manic depression can worsen psoriasis

✓ Sunlight can aggravate the condition as well as relieve it

Types of psoriasis

You may find that your psoriasis comes and goes and disappears for months or years at a time. You may even have only one episode during your lifetime. The condition may start slowly, with just a few patches, or much more explosively, especially after a sore throat caused by the bacterium *Streptococcus*.

Psoriasis is usually easy for doctors to diagnose. However, it can be mistaken for other skin conditions. In elderly people, for example, psoriasis is often confused with eczema. Eczema and psoriasis are both common disorders, and you may even suffer from the two conditions at the same time.

ECZEMA VERSUS PSORIASIS

Eczema is also known as dermatitis and typically causes a dry, irritated skin. It exists in a variety of forms, including an inherited tendency to a group of allergic conditions (atopic eczema) such as eczema, asthma and hayfever and irritation of the skin after exposure to certain chemicals (contact dermatitis).

The word eczema literally means 'to boil'. In the initial stages of the condition, your skin can look as if has been boiled, with a red appearance and tiny blisters. This is usually followed by dryness and scaling – it is at this stage that eczema can be mistaken for psoriasis.

Elderly people are prone to dry skin and eczema and it is often impossible to decide whether their rash is the result of eczema or psoriasis or both – even a biopsy may not be conclusive. It is important to discover the cause of the rash, because some of the topical treatments for psoriasis can irritate skin affected by eczema.

In young adults, it can be difficult to distinguish between psoriasis and seborrhoeic dermatitis. Seborrhoeic dermatitis is

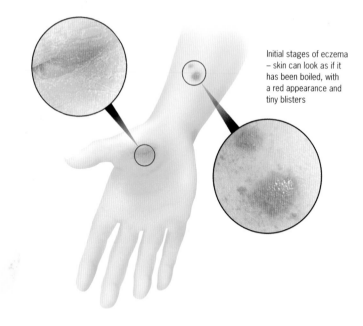

Later eczema typically dries and scales, and is often confused with psoriasis

Initial stages of eczema – skin can look as if it has been boiled, with a red appearance and tiny blisters

Eczema is also known as dermatitis and typically causes a dry, irritated skin. Psoriasis is often confused with eczema.

a form of eczema that produces a scaly scalp and characteristic rash on the face and trunk. It is caused at least in part by an infection with a yeast called *Pityrosporum*. Seborrhoeic dermatitis typically affects the front of the scalp, eyebrows, outer part of the ears, the sides of the nose, laughter lines around the mouth, and under the arms, breast and groin. It also causes irritation of the eyes.

Psoriasis may be confused with seborrhoeic dermatitis because psoriasis can affect the same areas of the body in its initial stages. The treatments for the conditions are different, so it is important to try to differentiate between the two, although sometimes only time will tell. The treatment for seborrhoeic dermatitis involves anti-fungal creams and hair preparations (Nizoral) and creams containing sulphur and salicyclic acid to help dampen down the inflammation. Seborrhoeic dermatitis, like psoriasis, can't be cured, but can be greatly improved.

PLAQUE PSORIASIS

This is the most common form of psoriasis. The individual plaques are not usually very itchy. They are, however, very red and covered with flaky silvery-white scales. If you scrape away the scales, with a fingernail, for example, the plaques may bleed.

The plaques usually have a clear edge, unlike most forms of eczema, and are usually symmetrical (one side of the body mirrors the other). The most common affected sites are the elbows, knees and scalp, but the plaques can occur anywhere on your body. Fortunately, the face is not commonly affected, although your forehead may be if your scalp is involved, with plaques appearing in front of your hairline.

The appearance of the plaques depends on where they are found on your body. In moist areas, such as the creases of the armpits and the groin,

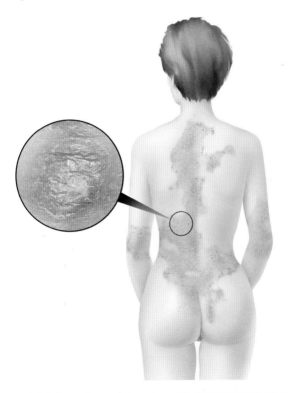

Plaque psoriasis is the most common form of psoriasis. Individual plaques are not usually very itchy. They are, however, very red and covered with flaky, silvery-white scales.

between the buttocks and under the breasts, there is little or no scaling – the patches are red with a sharp border. The palms and soles, however, tend to be scaly, but, because the skin is much thicker at these sites, the colour of the plaques is much less red. In most people, the plaques are large, often several centimetres or more across. Occasionally, people have several much smaller lesions of up to one centimetre.

The appearance of the plaques may be improved by topical treatments, especially the prolonged application of strong corticosteroids. When the plaques look angry and red, they can form little blisters (pustules), and this is often referred to as 'unstable psoriasis'. Short-contact dithranol or tar preparations are usually used to treat stable plaque psoriasis. Unstable psoriasis, however, many require hospital admission. The broad outlook, as for all types of psoriasis, is that there is no overall cure, but treatments can be very effective.

GUTTATE PSORIASIS

Guttate psoriasis usually occurs in children or young adults, and often follows a severe sore throat or bout of tonsillitis caused by a streptococcal infection. The sore throat is followed 7 to 14 days later by the sudden appearance of plaques of psoriasis all over the body, especially on the trunk and limbs. The plaques are small, usually less than one centimetre in diameter. Itching is usually mild or absent. This type of psoriasis has

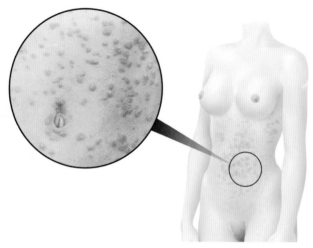

Guttate psoriasis is characterised by the sudden appearance of tiny plaques of psoriasis, possibly all over the body, but especially on the trunk and limbs.

an excellent outlook, and usually settles within a few weeks or months with topical treatments. Sometimes, a short course of ultraviolet light is also helpful.

Pustular psoriasis

Pustular psoriasis usually exists as a large red area covered with green tender pustules (blisters) that are one to two millimetres in diameter. Despite their colour, the pustules are not infected. The green colour is caused by masses of white blood cells called polymorph leucocytes. These cells flood into any part of the skin that is inflamed or damaged to try to fight off infection and to aid recovery. After 7 to 10 days, the pustules become dispersed and a brown scale appears. This brown scale is shed as further pustules develop elsewhere, often in a continuous cycle.

In the most common form of pustular psoriasis, the palms and soles are involved. Unlike eczema covering these areas, the psoriasis tends to be sore rather than itchy. Pustular psoriasis is uncomfortable and unsightly, and can make writing or walking difficult. The treatment involves the use of strong steroid creams such as Betnovate. This type of psoriasis usually improves within a few weeks, but may recur months, or even years, later.

A less common form of pustular psoriasis occurs when ordinary plaques of psoriasis start to blister. This can happen spontaneously,

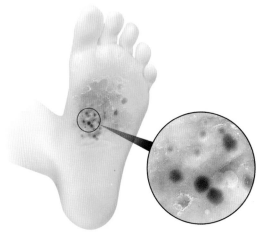

Pustular psoriasis usually exists as a large red area covered with green tender pustules (blisters) that are one to two millimetres in diameter.

but is more likely to follow the long-term use of strong topical corticosteroid treatments.

The most severe – and fortunately the most rare – form is called generalised pustular psoriasis. A patient becomes ill and feverish, and there is a sudden onset of tiny pustules all over the skin, usually starting on the upper trunk but spreading all over within hours or days. This requires hospital admission. Generalised pustular psoriasis can occur in people who already have psoriasis, but it sometimes occurs in people without this medical history. Occasionally, the pustular change is induced by the over-use of strong topical corticosteroid applications.

ERYTHRODERMA

This is fortunately a rare event, but can be serious and even life threatening in elderly people. It can even occur in someone without a history of psoriasis. In people with erythroderma, their skin becomes red and hot and continually scales. They lose their ability to control their body temperature and lose heat, body fluids and protein. Inpatient treatment is essential, and involves supportive measures, such as attaching an intravenous drip to replace the lost body fluids and applying soothing products and weak steroid creams. Full recovery is possible, although the outlook depends on the severity of the condition, overall health of the person affected and speed of treatment.

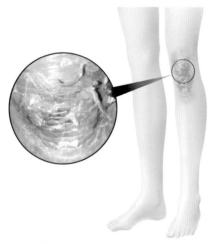

In erythroderma the skin becomes red hot and continually scales. The patient loses the ability to control body temperature, losing heat, fluids and protein.

NAPKIN PSORIASIS

Psoriasis in babies is rare. Most rashes that occur in the nappy area are caused by eczema, a fungus called *Candida* (thrush) or the irritant effect of urine. However, occasionally a red rash with a sharp border occurs and looks like psoriasis. Some babies can develop plaque psoriasis on their elbows and knees. Nappy rash is initially treated with an anti-fungal cream (Canesten) or an anti-fungal and steroid combination (Canesten-HC). The likelihood of the baby developing psoriasis later in life is increased, although not inevitable, and needs to be discussed with a specialist.

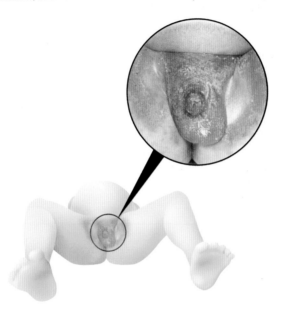

Psoriasis in babies is rare but occasionally a red rash with a sharp border occurs, called napkin psoriasis or nappy rash.

LINEAR PSORIASIS

Most psoriasis is symmetrical and widespread. But very occasionally, someone with plaque psoriasis has only the red patches and white scaling in a line down one limb or possibly on the trunk. This linear or naevoid type of psoriasis needs to be distinguished from other linear rashes, such as an epidermal naevus (birthmark) or an unusual form of eczema. A biopsy will usually show the typical changes of psoriasis under the microscope. The treatment and outlook are the same as for plaque psoriasis.

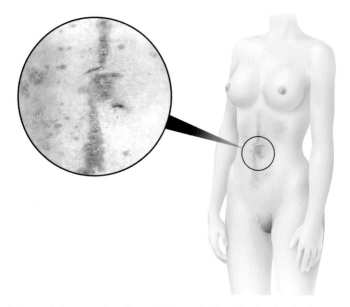

Linear psoriasis occurs where the red patches and white scaling form in a line down one limb or on the trunk.

PLAQUE PSORIASIS AT DIFFERENT SITES
Scalp

The scalp is a very common site for psoriasis and you may find that it is the only area involved. Usually, psoriasis on the scalp consists of clear-edged patches that are red, scaly and often lumpy. Hair is not usually affected. Scalp psoriasis is quite unlike seborrhoeic dermatitis, which has much more diffuse scaling, no lumpiness and no well-defined patches. Moreover, psoriasis often extends beyond the hairline. Sometimes psoriasis starts off looking like seborrhoeic dermatitis before evolving into more typical psoriasis.

The treatment of scalp psoriasis involves oily preparations with three per cent salicylic acid to reduce scaling (for example, Meted). You rub these preparations into your scalp three times a week, then wash them out with tar shampoo (for example, Clinitar) four to six hours later. You may even find that a combined salicylic acid and tar combination, such as Cocois, is sufficient. Vitamin D derivatives, such as Dovonex, can also be useful. Good short-term results can be obtained by using steroid scalp applications such as Betnovate, but these aren't as effective in the long term.

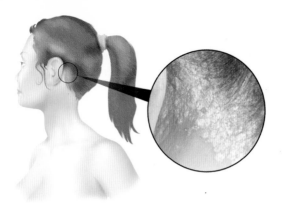

The scalp is a very common site for psoriasis, consisting of clear-edged patches that are red, scaly and often lumpy.

Flexures (creases)

You may find that psoriasis occurs where your skin creases, such as in your armpits, under your breasts, in your groin, between your buttocks and on your genitalia. As these sites are very moist, the plaques lose their scales and tend to be red with a sharp border. You may find the psoriasis is sore, especially while you are moving around.

The treatment is a combination of anti-fungal and steroid creams, such as Canesten-HC. The outlook is the same as for plaque psoriasis, although

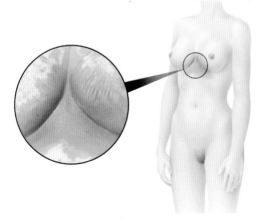

Psoriasis often occurs where your skin creases, such as under the armpits and breasts, in the groin, between your buttocks and on the genitalia.

flexure psoriasis may be particularly obstinate to treat because it can be difficult to get creams to stay in place without being rubbed off. In addition, the constant chafing that may occur in the skin creases (under heavy breasts, for example) can make it hard for the skin to recover.

Palms and soles

When plaque psoriasis occurs on the palms and soles, the patches are less red with thicker, more adherent scale than in plaque psoriasis elsewhere on the body, where the scale is much finer and flakes off easily. Sometimes, the skin's surface is cracked. If your fingertips are involved, it can be quite sore. Treatment is with moisturisers (E45, for example) and steroid creams, but the same problems seen with psoriasis in the flexures can occur and may delay healing.

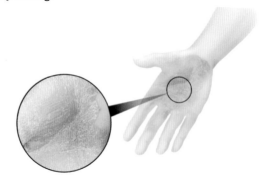

Plaque psoriasis on the palms.

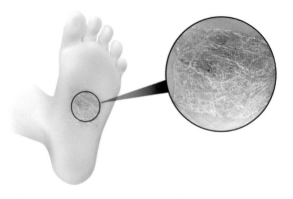

Plaque psoriasis on the soles.

Mouth

Psoriasis rarely, if ever, involves the mucous membrane (the membrane lining the mouth). However, in severe cases, the tongue can be involved, producing a characteristic pattern called the 'geographical tongue'. This is usually without symptoms. Geographical tongue often occurs in people who have no skin disease of any kind, but has also been noted in generalised pustular psoriasis.

Köbner plaque psoriasis

Sometimes psoriasis occurs in injured skin, most commonly appearing as a line in an operation scar or in scratches. Occasionally, it develops in the spots produced by chickenpox. Some other skin diseases can also be triggered in this way, but this is particularly common with psoriasis. Once triggered, the rash looks the same as before, but stays in lines, although the plaques may enlarge and look typical of plaque psoriasis, especially after chickenpox. The phenomenon of Köbner psoriasis may be associated with more conventional psoriasis at the usual sites. This type of psoriasis often heals on its own.

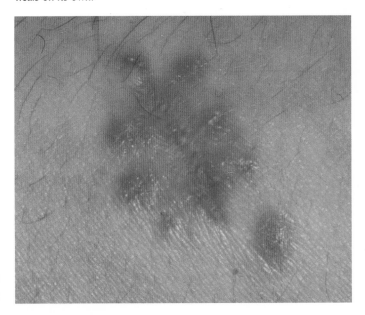

Köbner plaque psoriasis – psoriasis occurring in injured skin, most commonly appearing as a line in an operation scar or in scratches.

Nails

The fingernails and toenails are commonly affected by psoriasis. The nails may be pitted or start to separate from the nail bed (a process called onycholysis). In onycholysis, the nail usually has a whitish appearance. It is possible to get either pitting or onycholysis without necessarily having psoriasis, but if you get both nail problems together, psoriasis is likely to be the cause. If the nail is severely damaged, it will become crumbly. It is important to exclude tinea (ringworm) as a cause by taking nail samples.

If you have psoriasis of the nails, you may notice that your nails grow more quickly than normal. Although the treatment of this form of psoriasis is extremely difficult, good nail care by a professional manicurist may help to disguise the appearance of your nails.

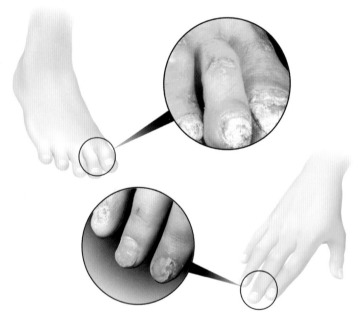

The fingernails and toes are often affected by psoriasis.

KEY POINTS

✓ Psoriasis comes and goes

✓ In elderly people, it is often mistaken for eczema

✓ The face is not commonly affected

✓ Guttate psoriasis may follow streptococcal tonsillitis

✓ The appearance of psoriasis depends on where the plaques are found

What treatments are available?

Not everyone with psoriasis wants to treat their symptoms. In fact, once you know what psoriasis is, you may be happy to live with the occasional flare-up of a few patches on your elbows and knees and just use self-help measures such as complementary therapies. You may want to get skin preparations over the counter (OTC), buying them at the pharmacy as and when you need them. This is fine, once the diagnosis has been made and you are satisfied that you can handle the treatment yourself.

Stronger treatments are only available on prescription; some of these are not usually prescribed by GPs, but only by a hospital skin specialist (dermatologist), although, once the dermatologist has started you off on the treatment, your GP may be able to take over. Treatments that are offered only in hospitals are usually systemic in action, which means that they don't just affect the skin, but affect the whole body.

The treatments will be discussed in this chapter under the following headings:

● Self-help: complementary therapies.

● Over-the-counter treatments (OTC): creams and ointments available over the counter from pharmacies.

● Prescription-only medicines (POM): topical treatments (applied to the skin or scalp) from your GP or dermatologist.

● Hospital treatments: systemic treatments – drugs taken by mouth or treatments that affect the whole body (for example, radiation treatments), usually from a dermatologist.

TREATMENTS FOR PSORIASIS

SELF-HELP
- Complementary therapies

OVER-THE-COUNTER TREATMENTS
- Moisturisers
- Tar products
- Very mild topical corticosteroids
- Salicylic acid products

PRESCRIPTION-ONLY MEDICINES (POM) AVAILABLE FROM A GP OR DERMATOLOGIST
- Moisturisers: may be cheaper on prescription than over the counter
- Topical corticosteroids
- Tar products
- Salicylic acid products
- Dithranol products
- Topical retinoids
- Vitamin D analogues

HOSPITAL TREATMENTS
- Ingram regimen
- PUVA – systemic
- Methotrexate – systemic
- Cyclosporin A – systemic

SELF-HELP

Complementary medicine

Many people with psoriasis try complementary therapies. This may be because conventional treatment has no effect on their psoriasis or because they are worried about the side effects of the treatments that they have been using. Undoubtedly, complementary treatments, such as acupuncture, homoeopathy and healing, can help some people. Relaxation therapies, such as yoga, are useful if stress is a common trigger of flare-ups. We don't know how all complementary therapies work. In fact, some may help simply because you believe that they will (the placebo effect). It is important to remember that not all complementary therapies are entirely without side effects; for example, herbal products, particularly Chinese herbal medicines, are not all well standardised and can cause side effects such as liver damage. If you wish to try complementary therapies for your psoriasis, make sure that you consult a properly qualified practitioner.

OVER-THE-COUNTER TREATMENTS

Moisturisers (emollients)

These are available on general sale in many outlets, for example, in supermarkets and over the counter at pharmacies. If you need large quantities of moisturisers, you may find it cheaper to get them on prescription from your GP.

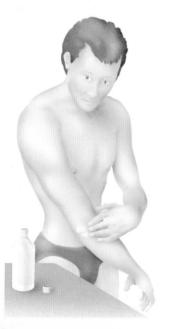

The regular use of emollients helps to relieve itching and scaling in psoriasis. Emollients smooth, soothe and hydrate the skin by sealing in moisture. Their effects tend to be short-lived, so they need to be applied regularly, perhaps three times a day. Light moisturisers, such as aqueous creams, are the easiest to use, but greasier preparations, such as emulsifying ointment BP, may be necessary for very dry skin or areas where cream gets rubbed off easily, such as the soles of the feet.

Emollients available over the counter include:

- Bath oil containing soya oil (Balneum bath oil)

- Creams containing liquid paraffin and white soft paraffin (E45)

- Creams containing glycerol (Neutrogena)

- Creams containing urea, which reduces scale (Nutraplus)

- Ointments (greasy) containing emulsifying ointment (Emulsifying ointment BP).

For many people with psoriasis, the loose silvery scale is the most embarrassing aspect of their condition, as flakes show up easily on clothes and carpet. A simple emollient can make the scale disappear, but it won't get rid of the plaques, which remain red. You can apply emollients directly onto your skin (creams or ointments), put them into the bath (oils) or use them in the shower (gels). They are all safe to use in the long term and will generally cause no side effects. Very occasionally, however, you may be sensitive to one of the ingredients (particularly lanolin) and will need to change to another cream if irritation occurs.

Tar products

There are numerous creams, ointments, bath products and scalp applications containing coal tar. Coal tar products (Alphosyl, Clinitar and Pragmatar, for example) reduce scaling and inflammation. They work by inhibiting DNA synthesis, which is necessary for cell multiplication, and therefore reduce the rapid turnover of skin cells.

Tar products have been available for many years. The original preparations could not be used on the face because they caused irritation, and many people disliked their strong, characteristic odour. However, newer products, such as Carbo-dome, have a milder odour and can be used over the whole body. Coal tar baths can be very soothing for people with widespread psoriasis and are part of the Ingram regimen.

Most tar products are available over the counter, but you should discuss their place in the treatment of your psoriasis with your GP or dermatologist before you use them. Tar cannot be used in sore or pustular psoriasis because it will cause severe irritation. Other possible side effects include an acne-like rash and skin, hair and fabric staining.

Mild topical corticosteroids (steroid creams and ointments)

You can buy weak topical corticosteroids (steroid preparations applied to the skin) over the counter as Dermacort, Hc45 and Lanacort. These preparations are available as creams or ointments and contain up to one per cent hydrocortisone, which is the weakest type of corticosteroid usually prescribed by doctors. Weak steroid creams may not have much effect on psoriasis and also have some drawbacks, so buying them over the counter is not really recommended. For more on topical corticosteroids, see 'Prescription-only medicines' below.

Salicylic acid

This is the active ingredient of aspirin, which helps to get rid of scaling. It may be combined in creams with tar (Pragmatar), dithranol (Dithranol paste BP) or tar and dithranol (Psorin). Although these creams have very few side effects, they may irritate or dry out your skin.

PRESCRIPTION-ONLY MEDICINES

Topical corticosteroids

These are steroid creams, ointments and lotions that are applied to the skin, rather than being taken orally as tablets. They have a vital role in the treatment of psoriasis because they work by damping down inflammation. You can buy weak steroids over the counter (see the previous section), but it is best to seek medical advice before using them as they can cause side effects.

For thick plaques of psoriasis, fairly potent corticosteroids are needed to gain benefit. However, these suppress the plaques, rather than clearing them completely. If topical corticosteroids are used constantly, a rebound reaction can occur – the plaques often worsen and may even change to pustular psoriasis. If potent corticosteroid preparations are used for many months, they can thin the skin permanently and even cause scars (called striae). In particular, potent corticosteroids should not be used on the face, in the flexures (creases) or on the genital area.

If potent corticosteroids are used over a widespread area of the body for prolonged periods, they may be absorbed in large-enough amounts to cause severe systemic side effects. These effects include high blood pressure, diabetes, thinning bones (osteoporosis) and Cushing's syndrome (a condition causing weight gain, a moon face and acne). These reactions are fortunately very rare, and potent corticosteroids are not prescribed for extensive areas of the body for prolonged periods.

Another problem that occurs if potent topical steroids are used continuously is that, over a period of time, they become less effective. The body gets used to the strength of the cream and requires ever more powerful strengths to achieve the same result. A break in treatment is often required for them to return to their full potency. This effect is called tachyphylaxis.

Topical corticosteroids do have considerable benefit in psoriasis, and weaker products such as hydrocortisone can be used on the face, in the flexures and on the genitals with little risk of skin damage. The weaker steroids work well at these sites because the plaques here are usually quite thin. In addition, the corticosteroid is effectively absorbed into the skin because more moisture is present.

Potent corticosteroids are tolerated quite well on the scalp without much skin thinning and are useful for mild scalp psoriasis. However, if

TOPICAL CORTICOSTEROIDS

Available over the counter:
Mild (suitable for all ages and all body sites)
- Hydrocortisone 1 per cent

Available on prescription only:
Moderately potent (still relatively safe and used at all sites, but best avoided on the face of children unless for short spells):
- Clobetasone butyrate 0.05 per cent
- Flurandrenolone 0.0125 per cent

Potent (can thin the skin; avoid as far as possible in children and don't use on the face; relatively safe in mild scalp psoriasis):
- Betamethasone valerate 0.1 per cent or 0.025 per cent
- Hydrocortisone butyrate
- Mometasone furoate 0.1 per cent
- Fluticasone propionate 0.05 per cent
- Beclomethasone dipropionate 0.025 per cent
- Betamethasone dipropionate 0.05 per cent
- Budesonide 0.025 per cent
- Fluocinolone acetonide 0.025 per cent

Very potent (great care required; use for only short spells and virtually never on the face; should probably be avoided altogether in children):
- Clobetasol propionate 0.05 per cent

the plaques are raised and lumpy, they need to be thinned by other means before corticosteroids have a chance to work.

Vitamin D analogues
These are the most important recent innovation in the treatment of psoriasis. They are available on prescription only and are usually offered by GPs rather than by a dermatologist. The analogues are available as calcipotriol cream, ointment and scalp solution, and tacalcitol ointment.

Vitamin D analogues are the treatment of choice for plaque psoriasis. In general, about one-third of patients do very well with almost complete clearing, one-third derive some benefit and one-third are not helped very much. The analogues work, at least in part, by causing the epidermal cells (keratinocytes) to divide in a more normal way and therefore produce normal keratin. They are relatively safe and can be used on children. Unlike topical corticosteroids, they do not thin the skin.

If excessive amounts of vitamin D analogues are used in very widespread psoriasis, a significant amount may be absorbed by the skin. This can increase the calcium content of the blood to very high levels, which can damage the kidneys and cause widespread problems. However, if you stick to 100 grams of 50-microgram strength calcipotriol, which is the usual prescribed weekly dose, you should not experience any problems. Vitamin D analogues can cause irritation, so don't get them in your eyes; use them with care in the creases of your skin and on your genitals, where the skin is more delicate.

Short-contact dithranol

Dithranol is a highly effective synthetic compound, available only on prescription in various products, including Dithrocream and Micanol. It is very effective in the treatment of chronic plaque psoriasis. It works by inhibiting the synthesis of DNA, therefore preventing the rapid cell turnover. The main problems with dithranol are that it tends to burn and irritate

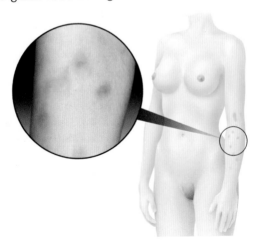

Dithranol is very effective in the treatment of chronic plaque psoriasis. However, it can burn and irritate normal skin, and stain the skin a purple–brown colour.

normal skin and can also stain the skin a purple–brown colour.

Almost 20 years ago, it was discovered that dithranol did not have to be left on the skin for 24 hours as previously thought; it could be removed after 10 to 30 minutes and still have a beneficial effect, but with much less staining and irritation. This short-contact dithranol treatment can be used by well-motivated patients at home under the supervision of their GP.

The products suitable for short-contact dithranol treatment come in five strengths: 0.1 per cent, 0.25 per cent, 0.5 per cent, 1 per cent and 2 per cent. Patients should start at the weakest and move up in strength every two to three days, unless irritation or soreness occurs. Although dithranol is in contact with the skin for 30 minutes (the usual time of application), it will stain any clothing permanently, and contact with soft furnishings should be avoided. When washed off the skin, dithranol tends to stain baths or showers and should be cleaned off immediately.

When dithranol is used correctly and carefully, about two-thirds of patients gain a satisfactory response, often with a remission lasting several months. The full Ingram regimen (see 'Hospital treatments') gives more complete and consistent results, but the short-contact method enables people to experience the benefits of dithranol at home. There is some evidence that, in the full Ingram regimen, the dithranol paste can be removed after two hours with the same results as leaving it on for 24 hours.

Topical retinoids

Topical retinoid creams are derived from vitamin A. Oral retinoids (described in 'Hospital treatments') are more powerful and more effective than the creams, but have far more side effects. Topical retinoids work by encouraging skin cells to mature properly, rather than dividing too rapidly and producing the poorly formed skin cells that make up the plaques. The major side effect is redness and skin peeling for several days after the cream is applied, but this usually settles with time.

The only topical retinoid used in psoriasis is tazarotene (Zorac). This was recently introduced for mild-to-moderate psoriasis that covers less than ten per cent of the body. A number of retinoids are also available for topical use in acne and various scaly disorders.

HOSPITAL TREATMENTS (DERMATOLOGY DEPARTMENTS)

If your psoriasis is proving difficult to treat with more standard treatments (such as those described previously), your GP will refer you to a hospital skin specialist (dermatologist). There are also a few rare instances in which a particularly severe form of psoriasis requires urgent hospital admission. The specific treatment you are given depends on the type and severity of your psoriasis and what you have already tried.

Dithranol (Anthralin) in the Ingram regimen

The use of short-contact dithranol is described in the previous section. Dithranol has been the standard hospital-based treatment in dermatology departments since the regimen was described by Professor Ingram in 1953. In many centres, it is used in outpatient units, but, in others, patients have to be admitted to hospital for treatment. The Ingram regimen involves lying in a warm bath containing a coal tar solution of 1 in 800. After drying off, you are exposed to ultraviolet UVB rays to redden your skin slightly. Dithranol is then applied to the plaques and the normal skin is protected as talc and gauze dressings are applied over the dithranol. The whole procedure is repeated daily.

If you attend an outpatient unit, you'll be treated five days a week; if you are an inpatient, you'll probably be treated seven days a week.

About 85 per cent of patients are free of their psoriasis after about 20 treatments, although some people's skin will clear much sooner. Treatments can be repeated if necessary, but the exposure to UVB rays has to be limited to avoid increasing the risk of skin cancer.

The advantage of dithranol over many other treatments is that it is well tried and tested, and is very safe. Once the patient is cleared with dithranol, he or she is likely to experience a period free of psoriasis ranging from four to six months, before the plaques gradually come back. Sometimes the remission lasts for one to two years.

The disadvantages of dithranol are that it is very time-consuming and rather messy. People in certain jobs find that it is difficult to continue working while using dithranol – for example, in manual labour, sweating may cause the dithranol to spread onto normal skin, where it may cause soreness. Dithranol may also be difficult for people who have to wear a suit for work.

There are two main side effects of dithranol: neither is serious, but both limit its use. Dithranol can stain the plaques and irritate and stain the surrounding skin. The purple–brown discoloration of the skin tends to peel off after a few days, but the staining of clothes, bathtubs and other objects touched by the skin may be permanent.

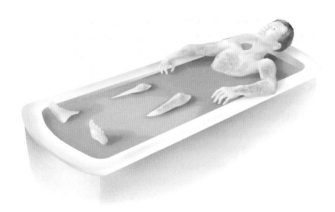

The patient lies in a warm bath containing a coal tar solution of 1 in 800.

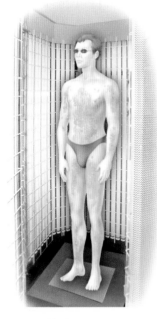

After drying off the patient is exposed to ultraviolet UVB rays to redden the skin slightly.

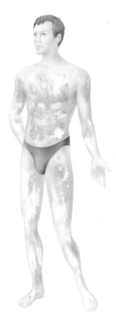

Dithranol is applied to the plaques which are then overlaid with gauze and talc, to protect the surrounding skin.

The Ingram regimen.

Irritation and burning of the surrounding skin can be controlled by beginning with the weakest concentration of dithranol and increasing the strength every one to two days. The starting concentration is usually about 0.05 per cent, gradually increasing up to three to five per cent in some patients.

As a result of the staining and possible soreness, attempts have been made to produce chemicals that still have similar benefits to dithranol but without these side effects. These attempts have not been very successful – the newer products tend to have fewer side effects but also seem to be less effective. To gain the full benefit from a 24-hour application of dithranol, staining almost always occurs, although the irritation and burning can be kept to a minimum by carefully adjusting the concentration according to the response.

Ultraviolet light

Most patients with psoriasis find that sunlight helps their condition. In fact, for many, one to two visits a year to a sunny climate will work wonders for their skin. The sun emits energy in the form of ultraviolet rays, which are invisible to the naked eye. These rays can be divided into three forms, depending on their wavelength: UVA (315 to 400 nanometres), UVB (280 to 315 nanometres) and UVC (100 to 280 nanometres). Most rays are UVA, which has the longest wavelength and penetrates deepest into the skin. UVB rays have a shorter wavelength and are more intense, but penetrate the skin less deeply. UVC rays are the shortest and are lost in the atmosphere before they reach Earth.

UVB phototherapy

UVB rays are the cause of sunburn. They are beneficial in psoriasis and can be artificially produced by sunlamps. The use of these sunlamps in psoriasis is called phototherapy.

Broad-band UVB phototherapy can be used on its own, particularly in guttate psoriasis. The treatment is usually given three times a week, although it can be given daily. However, UVB phototherapy is more usually combined with dithranol in the Ingram regimen or with tar in the Goeckerman regimen. It can also be used in conjunction with oral retinoid drugs (acitretin) or with topical vitamin D analogues (calcipotriol or tacalcitol).

TL-01: narrow-band UV at 311 nanometres

Phillips recently devised lamps that seem to be more effective than broad-band UVB at clearing psoriasis. These narrow-band lamps are gradually taking over, as hospitals replace their broad-band UVB units. The narrow-band UV lamps can also be used with other treatments as mentioned under UVB phototherapy.

The Psoriasis Treatment Centre at the Dead Sea, in Israel, reports that three-quarters of patients improved by 90 per cent or more after four weeks of treatment. It is likely that UVB rays are the main reason for this benefit.

Psoralens and UVA photochemotherapy (PUVA)

Certain chemicals from plants (especially from *Ammi majus*) called psoralens seem to benefit psoriasis if they are used after the skin has been irradiated with long-wave UVA light. The psoralens are most effective when they are taken orally, although they can also be used on the skin itself or in the bath.

The interaction of psoralens with UVA is known as PUVA or photochemotherapy, and has been used since the mid-1970s. PUVA is a highly effective treatment for widespread plaque psoriasis. In some centres, the psoralen is taken orally two hours before UVA exposure, and in other units, it is added to a bath that is taken immediately before UVA exposure. There are two types of psoralens used in PUVA treatment. Some patients experience nausea after taking 8-methoxypsoralen. If this is the case, 5-methoxypsoralen – a different, equally effective form that doesn't have this side effect – can be used.

In most centres, the treatment is undertaken twice a week. About 90 per cent of patients will clear completely in six to eight weeks. During treatment, the skin usually becomes tanned. The clearance that results will last, on average, for four to six months before the psoriasis gradually returns. However, in some patients, the psoriasis may come back straight away whereas, in others, it will take years to return.

PUVA is most effective in widespread plaque psoriasis, but it can be used in pustular psoriasis (generalised and localised, involving the palms and soles), and in erythroderma. However, in these types of psoriasis, there are alternative treatments that may be more effective. PUVA is not effective in the scalp or flexures.

In many centres, a retinoid drug (acitretin) is given for ten days before PUVA and continued right through the PUVA course. It has been shown that only about half the exposure to UVA is required when the treatment is combined in this way.

The immediate side effect from PUVA is burning from the UVA rays, so the starting dose of UVA is usually low and is then increased gradually. There has been anxiety that, in oral PUVA, where the psoralen is taken by mouth, cataracts may develop. There has, however, been no clinical evidence of this, although, as some initial reports suggested the possibility, patients are all required to wear special protective glasses from the moment they take the drug and for the rest of that day. They are also required to wear special protective goggles while in the UVA treatment unit.

The main concern with PUVA is an increased risk of the development of skin cancers. This is a dose-related effect, so the more exposure to UVA the greater the risk. Fortunately, the risk is largely of the relatively easily treated non-melanoma skin cancer and not melanoma itself. Patients who have had high-dose PUVA (more than 300 treatments) have a sixfold increased risk of developing skin cancer when compared with low-dose PUVA patients (less than 160 treatments). Fair-skinned people have twice the risk of skin cancer compared with dark-skinned people.

Recent guidelines from the British Association of Dermatologists and the Royal College of Physicians suggest that the lifetime maximum of PUVA treatment should not exceed 1,000 joules per square centimetre (J/cm^2) if at all possible. This is the equivalent of about 100 PUVA treatments or about six to eight courses. However, for people who find that PUVA is effective, once they have had 1,000 J/cm^2 of energy of UVA, there would need to be a full discussion as to the relative risks of continuing further PUVA or switching to alternative treatments, which may also have side effects.

The risk of skin cancers appears to be greater on the male genitalia and therefore these should be covered during treatment. The face should also be covered unless it is affected by psoriasis, to prevent additional photoageing of the skin. There is no evidence that bath PUVA has less risk of skin cancer, but eye protection is not necessary as very little psoralen is absorbed.

Methotrexate

Methotrexate is an anti-mitotic (anti-cancer) drug and has been used extensively for psoriasis for more than 30 years. It inhibits DNA synthesis, and so slows down the epidermal cell turnover. Methotrexate works to a certain extent on all rapidly dividing cells, including blood cells, so regular blood counts are important to ensure that there are no adverse effects on the blood. Methotrexate may also affect the immune system abnormalities found in the skin of people with psoriasis.

Methotrexate is mainly used for severe, resistant psoriasis in elderly people who cannot manage other systemic treatments. It is highly effective in plaque psoriasis and is well tolerated; it also has a role in psoriatic erythroderma, generalised pustular psoriasis, psoriatic arthritis and pustular psoriasis of the palms and soles.

Methotrexate is usually given orally, but can also be given by intramuscular injections in some centres. The dose varies from 5 to 25 milligrams per week, although it is usually between 10 and 15 milligrams a week. Methotrexate is usually given as a single weekly dose, rather than several daily doses, as the side effects on the liver (see below) are reduced when the drug is given in this way.

Side effects of methotrexate
● **Nausea:** This is not usually a problem, but is occasionally the reason for stopping treatment.

● **Blood:** Methotrexate may cause bone marrow suppression, which can lead to anaemia, bruising and an inability to fight off infections properly. As a result of this, regular blood tests are required (usually weekly at first).

● **Liver:** Methotrexate can produce potentially serious and irreversible liver damage. However, when used in low doses and given weekly, the risk is low. Moreover, if alcohol intake is kept to a minimum, so as not to put a strain on the liver (not more than one to two units of alcohol a week), liver damage is rare. The liver function is checked regularly with a blood test.

Unfortunately, the liver can be damaged considerably by methotrexate before the blood tests reveal any abnormalities, because these tests are not always sensitive enough. In many centres, therefore, intermittent liver biopsies are performed, so that early damage can be identified and methotrexate treatment stopped if necessary. Liver biopsies involve putting a needle into the liver to extract a small sample of cells for examination under a microscope. Many centres will perform a liver biopsy before starting methotrexate or once a patient has been cleared of psoriasis, and then every few years while they remain on methotrexate.

The necessity of liver biopsies is under debate. Most centres still do biopsies in patients aged under 65 to make sure that their liver is not being damaged. Rheumatologists, however, use methotrexate extensively for rheumatoid arthritis and most do not do liver biopsies. Liver biopsy is relatively safe, although it is an invasive test that can cause some internal bleeding, pain and a small risk of infection. It is performed under ultrasound imaging control to keep complications to a minimum.

- **Effects on unborn children:** Methotrexate is a teratogen, which means that it can damage a developing baby if it is given to a pregnant woman. Therefore, women should not become pregnant while taking the drug. Men on methotrexate should also take care not to get a woman pregnant, because the drug can pass into the sperm and damage the fetus.

- **Kidney function:** Methotrexate does not damage the kidneys, although it is excreted (removed from the body) by them. It is important to check kidney function with a blood test at the start of treatment. If patients are on methotrexate for many years, annual blood checks are essential. Kidney function slowly deteriorates with age. If it is not checked regularly, methotrexate levels may rise in the blood and cause more side effects on the bone marrow and the liver. It may be necessary to reduce the methotrexate dose as years go by.

- **Drug interactions:** Methotrexate can interact with other drugs – it can make another drug more toxic by increasing its blood levels. This is particularly common with aspirin and other non-steroidal anti-inflammatory drugs. Therefore, if you are taking methotrexate, tell your doctor or pharmacist, so that he or she can assess the risk of drug interactions.

Hydroxyurea

Hydroxyurea is also an anti-cancer drug. It is much less popular than methotrexate but has a role in the treatment of psoriasis because it is moderately effective and does not damage the liver. Hydroxyurea is more likely, however, to cause bone marrow depression, so blood tests need to be performed more frequently than with methotrexate. Patients may also have a slightly lowered white blood cell count. Hydroxyurea is often best used in conjunction with the retinoid drug acitretin. It is given in a daily oral dose of between 0.5 and 1.5 grams. As with methotrexate, women should not get pregnant, and men should not father children, while taking hydroxyurea.

Oral retinoids

Retinoids are vitamin A drugs with the chemical name of tretinoin or isotretinoin. Acitretin is the main retinoid used in the treatment of psoriasis and is taken orally in a dose of 25 to 50 milligrams a day.

Retinoids have many effects on the skin. In particular, they promote epithelial cell differentiation, which means that they encourage skin cells in the epidermis to mature properly instead of reaching the skin's surface before they are fully formed.

On its own, acitretin is often only partially effective in plaque psoriasis. It is, however, particularly effective in generalised pustular psoriasis, erythrodermic psoriasis, pustular psoriasis of the palms and soles, and in unstable forms of psoriasis. Acitretin is often combined with other treatments such as PUVA, UVB phototherapy or hydroxyurea, and can also be combined with topical treatments such as vitamin D analogues. Acitretin can be used in children.

Side effects of oral retinoids

- **General:** The skin often becomes dry and the lips may crack. The eyes and nose may become dry too. Occasionally, hair loss occurs, although this reverses once the drug has been stopped.

- **Cholesterol and triglycerides:** Retinoid drugs tend to raise cholesterol and triglyceride levels in the body, so these will need to be checked occasionally. It is worthwhile controlling your intake of dairy products while on retinoids to reduce the chance of an elevation of your blood lipids.

- **Liver:** Very rarely, acitretin or retinoids cause inflammation of the liver (hepatitis).

- **Bony and soft tissue changes:** These changes are usually without symptoms and are therefore picked up only on an X-ray. Calcification may occur in the anterior spinal ligament. Other X-ray changes can occur but are of doubtful clinical significance.

- **Teratogenicity:** Women on retinoids must not get pregnant for two years after the course has been completed, as retinoids can cause birth defects. Although most of the acitretin is promptly excreted, it can be bound in fat for up to two years. The chance of having an abnormal child if a woman takes acitretin during pregnancy is extremely high. Men can father children while taking acitretin.

Cyclosporin A

Cyclosporin is developed from a fungus called *Tolypocladium inflatum gams*. It is an immunosuppressive drug and is used to control and prevent rejection of transplanted organs. In small doses, cyclosporin A is very effective in controlling psoriasis, probably by affecting the T cells, rather than by preventing the division of skin cells and their rapid turnover. Cyclosporin is given daily in doses of approximately three to five milligrams per kilogram of bodyweight (150 to 400 milligrams) orally in two divided doses. Cyclosporin A is well tolerated.

Side effects of cyclosporin A

● **Excess hairiness:** Unusual in the low doses that are used.

● **Gum:** Thickening of the gums may occur, but this is unusual in the low doses used.

● **Gout:** Occasionally, cyclosporin A can elevate uric acid levels, causing gout.

● **Renal function:** Although cyclosporin A is used in renal transplant recipients, it can actually damage the kidneys. This needs to be monitored by monthly blood tests. The drug is discontinued if tests show that renal function has altered by certain recognised parameters.

● **Hypertension:** A rise in blood pressure can occur with cyclosporin A so it is important that the blood pressure is checked monthly. Hypertension is independent of its effect on the kidneys. A mild elevation of the blood pressure does not mean that cyclosporin A has to be discontinued – treatment for the blood pressure can be introduced if necessary.

● **Long-term use of cyclosporin A:** Long-term use can lead to skin cancers so it is particularly important that people on cyclosporin A are given advice about sun protection.

● **Other considerations:** If you are taking cyclosporin A, you need to be wary of taking other oral drugs at the same time, as drug interactions can occur. For example, anti-inflammatory drugs, such as Brufen or Voltarol, which are used for aches and pains, can increase the amount of cyclosporin in your blood. This is because your kidneys' ability to get rid of the cyclosporin is diminished by the anti-inflammatories. If you are on cyclosporin, make sure that your doctors and pharmacist are aware of this before they try to prescribe/dispense another medicine for you.

A new drug called tacrolimus has recently been developed. Tacrolimus is similar to cyclosporin A. At present, it is under intensive study as an immunosuppressant in patients who receive a transplant and in those with psoriasis. There is hope that it may be used topically, as well as orally, but with fewer side effects than cyclosporin A.

TREATMENT OF DIFFERENT TYPES OF PSORIASIS
Scalp psoriasis

The treatment of scalp psoriasis is not always easy. For mild cases, in which the plaques are not lumpy or very scaly, a tar shampoo may be all that is required. Topical corticosteroids are often effective and the hairy scalp seems to tolerate them quite well without much thinning of the skin. However, they should not be used continuously.

For more severe psoriasis of the scalp with many lumpy lesions, the treatment is more difficult. The first thing is to remove the scale and so flatten the lesions. This can be done with salicylic acid products, of which there are many formulations. These products are often combined with tar, so they can be messy to use. However, if they are massaged well into the scalp and left on for some time (preferably hours), they will gradually remove all the scale, with the hair left intact. Another option is to use arachis oil, which is possibly less messy and non-smelly. Afterwards, the choices to keep the psoriasis from building up again include topical corticosteroids, vitamin D analogues (calcipotriol scalp solution) or possibly just a tar shampoo. Most patients with scalp psoriasis can keep it under reasonable control, but it is often difficult to clear it completely. It is not usually severe enough, however, to consider systemic treatment with agents such as methotrexate, retinoids or cyclosporin A. PUVA is of no help if the scalp is hairy.

Nail psoriasis

There is no treatment that is effective when used topically for nail psoriasis. If a patient has severe enough psoriasis elsewhere to warrant systemic treatment, then the nails may improve.

Pustular forms of psoriasis

Pustular psoriasis is most common on the palms and soles, but can occasionally occur in a severe form of generalised pustular psoriasis.

● **Localised pustular psoriasis on the palms and soles:** This can be very difficult to treat. Topical corticosteroids are ineffective, unless very potent products are used with the risk that thinning of the skin may occur. Dithranol is usually ineffective and is messy to use at these sites. Vitamin D analogues are only occasionally effective. For mild cases, moisturisers with the occasional use of a potent topical corticosteroid or possibly a vitamin D analogue are the best options. For the more severe forms, PUVA, methotrexate, hydroxyurea, with or without acitretin, and cyclosporin A are all helpful. However, potential side effects of these agents have to be balanced against the severity of the disorder.

● **Generalised pustular psoriasis:** Acitretin, cyclosporin A, methotrexate and occasionally PUVA are all effective in this rare form of psoriasis.

PSORIASIS AT DIFFERENT AGES

It can be very hard for parents to cope with seeing their children distressed because of a skin condition. Any child with an obvious skin problem may be subjected to teasing or even bullying, and parents and teachers must be particularly vigilant in looking out for this. It is worth talking to their head and class teacher to ensure that the pupils and teachers understand that psoriasis is not infectious. The Psoriasis Association can be particularly helpful in putting children with psoriasis in touch with others with the condition. It is also vital that your child understands his or her own condition and treatments, and that the explanation that you give is appropriate for the age. You may want to do this together with professionals in the field.

Most children with psoriasis will respond to topical vitamin D drugs, short-contact dithranol or long-contact dithranol, all with or without UVB phototherapy. Most doctors are reluctant to use PUVA in children because there is an upper limit of lifetime exposure to UVA rays to prevent an increased risk of skin cancer.

Fortunately, plaque psoriasis is rarely so severe in children that systemic treatments such as methotrexate, retinoids and cyclosporin A are required. Methotrexate is very rarely used in children because of the increased risk of liver damage with cumulative doses. Doctors are also reluctant to use prolonged courses of potent topical corticosteroids in children because of the thinning effect on the skin and possible formation of striae (streaks on the skin).

In elderly patients, it is important to remember that eczema and psoriasis are often confused. It is also essential to be particularly careful when using dithranol, topical retinoids or vitamin D drugs because they can all irritate the skin. Moisturisers are often very helpful and can be used in conjunction with topical corticosteroid ointments. A mild-to-moderate strength corticosteroid will often be adequate.

In elderly patients with widespread psoriasis, doctors often choose to use methotrexate, PUVA, hydroxyurea or cyclosporin A, especially if such a patient would find it difficult to attend an outpatient treatment unit on a regular daily basis.

KEY POINTS

✓ Complementary medicine has a role in some patients

✓ Some people with psoriasis are happy to use simple moisturisers

✓ Vitamin D analogues are the treatment of choice for mild-to-moderate psoriasis treated in general practice

✓ Potent topical corticosteroids should be used with great care and never for long courses

✓ Dithranol is the mainstay of hospital treatment and if used in a short-contact form produces less staining and burning than the long-contact form

✓ TL-01 narrow-band UV is superior to standard UVB phototherapy

✓ The risk of skin cancer after PUVA rises after about six to eight courses of treatment

✓ Methotrexate is perhaps the best systemic treatment for psoriasis

✓ Pustular psoriasis of the palms and soles is difficult to treat

✓ The scalp can be very resistant to treatment

Will the psoriasis come back?

Psoriasis tends to be a chronic condition that comes and goes. There may be long gaps when you have little or no skin problems at all. The best outlook seems to be after an episode of guttate psoriasis following streptococcal tonsillitis. A short course of UVB phototherapy with or without vitamin D analogues will often lead to remission that lasts for many years.

The pattern with typical plaque psoriasis is much more variable. The treatments most likely to induce a remission, rather than just suppress the psoriasis, are dithranol, UVB phototherapy and PUVA. With other treatments, psoriasis tends to return quite quickly. Topical corticosteroids and vitamin D analogues, for example, may suppress your psoriasis but are unlikely to induce a lasting remission.

In some people, after their psoriasis has been completely cleared they have many months or even years free from symptoms; in others, their psoriasis returns almost immediately and needs another course of treatment. If their psoriasis is severe enough, these people tend to require continuous systemic treatment such as methotrexate, hydroxyurea, retinoids or cyclosporin A. In one study, three out of 260 patients were clear of their psoriasis for more than five years after successful treatment, but most patients were not clear for more than six months.

Usually, the same treatment that previously caused the remission will do so again. But, sometimes, treatments lose their efficacy after several courses. This is particularly common with the Ingram regimen using dithranol and UVB phototherapy. The Ingram regimen can work well for many years giving remissions of several months, then either it suddenly stops clearing a patient or the remission becomes increasingly short, indicating that systemic treatment should be started.

KEY POINTS

✓ Psoriasis tends to be a continuing condition, the severity of which comes and goes

✓ Successful treatments vary in efficacy – ranging from a mild suppression of the psoriasis to complete remission that lasts for many years

✓ Usually, the treatment that previously caused a remission will do so again, but sometimes treatments lose their efficacy after several courses

Psoriasis and other diseases + lifestyle issues

PSORIATIC ARTHRITIS

Sometimes, people with psoriasis experience pain and swelling of some of their joints, typically the ends of their fingers and toes. When psoriasis and arthritis occur together, the resulting condition is called psoriatic arthritis.

The true incidence of psoriatic arthritis is unknown, because it depends on which population of psoriatic patients is investigated. In a hospital setting (where more severe psoriasis is likely to be under study) the prevalence of arthritis in patients with psoriasis is six to eight per cent (compared with 0.7 per cent in a control group with other skin diseases). Psoriatic arthritis is more common in women than in men, with a peak onset in the 40- to 60-year age group. Psoriasis starts before the arthritis in 65 per cent of cases, whereas the arthritis precedes the psoriasis in 19 per cent of cases; they occur at about the same time in 16 per cent.

There are several different patterns of psoriatic arthritis:

- You may find that the small joints of your fingers and toes are affected, particularly if you have severe nail psoriasis – this is the classic and typical psoriatic arthritis, and tends to occur only in people with psoriasis.

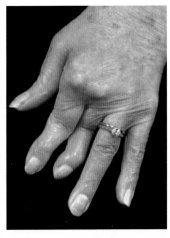

Psoriatic arthritis of the finger joints.

- You may have a rheumatoid arthritis pattern in your hands and feet. A blood test can help to differentiate between rheumatoid arthritis and psoriatic arthritis. In rheumatoid arthritis, a specific chemical in the blood known as rheumatoid factor is high, whereas, in psoriatic arthritis, it is low.

- You may get one or several joints involved on either side of your body. This may be the result of a rare form of particularly debilitating arthritis in which joints of your fingers and toes become permanently deformed and are unable to function.

- You may have arthritis of the spine, characterised by a stiff, painful lower back with pain on both sides where the sacro-iliac joint (at the back of your pelvis) is found.

TREATMENT

The treatment of psoriatic arthritis is similar to the management of rheumatoid arthritis. A variety of drugs is used.

- Non-steroidal anti-inflammatory drugs (NSAIDs), which suppress inflammation and relieve the pain and swelling of the joints. NSAIDs do not halt the progression of the disease. They are called 'non-steroidal' to distinguish them from corticosteroids, which also have anti-inflammatory properties.

- Sulphasalazine (a sulphur-based drug) and gold compounds, which dampen down inflammation and halt the progress of joint diseases.

- Methotrexate, which interferes with cell division and slows down the epidermal cell turnover.

- Azathioprine, an immunosuppressive drug that dampens down inflammation associated with arthritis.

- Cyclosporin A, which also suppresses the immune system and treats both the psoriasis and the arthritis.

OUTLOOK

Psoriatic arthritis usually causes less pain and disability than rheumatoid arthritis. It may improve dramatically with treatment, although the joint problems may recur at any time without warning. The outcome may be very hard to predict.

HIV AND AIDS

Occasionally, patients with AIDS develop particularly severe psoriasis. Many of the treatments for psoriasis, such as methotrexate,

PUVA and cyclosporin A, may not be suitable, because immunosuppressive therapy is harmful to these already immunocompromised patients. Retinoids and zidovudine (AZT) are both effective drugs and safer to use.

PSORIASIS IN RELATION TO ALCOHOL, SMOKING AND DIET

There appears to be a link between excessive alcohol intake and psoriasis. Research shows that men with psoriasis are more likely to be heavy drinkers than the rest of the male population, but this does not seem to be the case among women. Whether excess alcohol could actually cause psoriasis in men is far from clear. It would be quite understandable if people with psoriasis turned to drink more than usual because of the stress of having an unpleasant skin condition.

In very high doses, alcohol damages the liver. Many of the systemic treatments for psoriasis are best avoided in liver disease patients (methotrexate, for example), so it is important that people with psoriasis keep their alcohol intake to sensible levels. Otherwise, many effective systemic agents that may have been able to control their psoriasis will not be suitable for them.

Smokers are at an increased risk of pustular psoriasis of the palms and soles and of chronic plaque psoriasis. This is thought to result from the harmful effects of smoking on the immune system.

The role of diet in psoriasis management seems to be of little importance, although eating a balanced diet with plenty of fresh fruit and vegetables will help to keep you in general good health. However, if a person is obese and psoriasis involves the flexures, then losing weight may help, because chafing of layers of fat under the belly or under heavy breasts may lead to particularly persistent plaques.

KEY POINTS

✓ Some patients with psoriasis also have joint problems; this can be the result of the psoriasis, in which case it is called psoriatic arthritis

✓ Psoriatic arthritis is more common in women than in men

✓ Psoriatic arthritis can improve dramatically with treatment

✓ Eating a balanced diet with plenty of fruit and vegetables will help your general health, and at the least will not worsen your psoriasis

Future research

Research continues around the world into the understanding of psoriasis and its treatment. Advances are likely to occur in the field of molecular genetics in the near future, although the actual genes associated with psoriasis may not be identified for some time.

It is probably unrealistic to hope to find a complete cure for psoriasis. However, an increased understanding of the effects of psoriasis on epidermal cell turnover and the immunological changes that occur will undoubtedly lead to more effective – and safer – treatments. For example, we can hopefully expect newer, less-irritant, vitamin D analogues and topical retinoids.

Work is already under way to investigate a new drug called tacrolimus. This drug is similar to cyclosporin A and has properties that control the immune system. It is of particular interest because it may be active when applied to the skin as well as when taken orally.

Work is in its infancy on the use of photodynamic treatment of psoriasis, where certain porphyrin chemicals are applied to the skin and then exposed to visible light from special lamps. This treatment is already being used for the treatment of non-melanoma skin cancers in some places around the world.

Questions & answers

● Why have I got psoriasis when no one else in my family has it?

Psoriasis tends to run in families, but there are also trigger factors that activate the condition. Some of these triggers are known and some are not. It is therefore possible that members of your family have 'carried' the psoriasis genes but the condition itself has never surfaced. Alternatively, a brief attack of psoriasis in a relative many years ago may have been forgotten.

● Will my children get psoriasis?

A child is at an increased risk of psoriasis if one of their parents has the condition. This risk is increased dramatically if both parents have psoriasis.

● Why have I got psoriasis now when I have never had it before?

To develop psoriasis, you have to have a specific gene. There are then certain triggers that activate the condition, such as streptococcal tonsillitis, hormonal factors, sunburn, certain drugs and possibly stress. The psoriasis may be triggered at any time, and may develop for no obvious reason.

● Is psoriasis infectious?

No.

● Can psoriasis be cured completely?

Often psoriasis does not return for months or even years after a course of treatment. It cannot, however, be cured in the sense of 'banished forever'.

● Can I get rid of my psoriasis?

Psoriasis can usually be successfully treated. Various treatments are available, both topical and systemic; the treatment you use will depend on the type and severity of your condition. Most treatments help to relieve psoriasis; some even clear it up for long periods of time.

● What will happen to my psoriasis if I become pregnant?

The effect of pregnancy on psoriasis is variable. Some women find that their psoriasis improves during pregnancy; others find that their condition worsens. If you are taking medication for your psoriasis make sure that you speak to your doctor before becoming pregnant, because some medicines can harm the fetus.

● Are there any drugs that make psoriasis worse?

Yes, some drugs can worsen existing psoriasis. In particular, psoriasis can be aggravated by lithium, which is given for manic depression, and by a course of oral corticosteroids taken for other chronic medical conditions. Occasionally, beta-blocker drugs used for heart disease or hypertension aggravate psoriasis too. Some anti-malarial drugs are said to worsen psoriasis but in practice rarely do so.

● Is psoriasis the result of stress?

In most cases, no. In some people, however, stress makes their psoriasis worse, but it is not the actual cause.

● Will I get arthritis?

Not necessarily. In one hospital-based study, about six to eight per cent of patients with psoriasis developed some form of psoriatic arthritis. The figures are probably much lower than this in real life because this study focused on people with severe symptoms – most patients with mild psoriasis do not go to hospital dermatology departments.

Case histories

CASE 1

A boy of seven has plaque psoriasis limited to his scalp, elbows and knees with just a few scattered plaques all over

He would be treated with moisturisers, topical vitamin D analogues, such as calcipotriol applied in cream or ointment form twice a day, or short-contact dithranol cream. His scalp could be treated with calcipotriol scalp solution or, if severe, a salicylic acid and tar product to reduce the scaling before the calcipotriol scalp solution is applied. The treatment will need to be supervised by his parents.

CASE 2

A girl of seven has very widespread psoriasis covering most of her body

She should be referred to a hospital dermatology department for consideration of dithranol treatment in the Ingram regimen or possibly the vitamin D analogue calcipotriol with or without UVB phototherapy.

CASE 3

A girl or young woman has guttate psoriasis 10 to 14 days after a nasty bout of tonsillitis

This type of psoriasis often settles after six to eight weeks of using moisturisers and calcipotriol. Short-contact dithranol is another possibility if her symptoms are severe. A short course of UVB phototherapy is often very effective, but this will require referral of the patient to a dermatology department.

CASE 4

A man has plaque psoriasis limited to a few areas of his body

Moisturisers will help to reduce scaling, and he may not want to bother with other treatments. If, however, he wants to be treated, a topical vitamin D product, such as calcipotriol, is the best to begin with, in cream or ointment form and applied twice a day. An alternative treatment would be short-contact dithranol.

Case 5

A woman has widespread plaque psoriasis covering most of her body

It is worth trying vitamin D analogues first – for example, calcipotriol used topically twice a day – but only if less than 100 grams a week is required. If this is ineffective or if more than 100 grams a week is required, she should be referred to a dermatology department for dithranol in the Ingram regimen with UVB phototherapy or calcipotriol with UVB phototherapy. PUVA or systemic drugs should be considered if her psoriasis is really severe, fails to respond to other treatments or, having responded, flares up quickly.

Case 6

A man has severe plaque psoriasis or pustular psoriasis on his palms and soles that interferes with his work and leisure activities

A short course of a very potent topical corticosteroid is justifiable, but it is likely that his condition will flare up again once the treatment is discontinued. He should be referred to a hospital dermatology department for consideration of PUVA or another systemic treatment. A topical steroid could be used while he is waiting for an appointment.

Case 7

An elderly woman has very itchy psoriasis – especially on her legs

Elderly people often suffer from eczema. Their skin is often very dry and cracked and psoriasis and eczema can often coexist, so it is important to check that psoriasis is the cause of the itching. She may find that using moisturisers in the bath or shower and on her skin brings some relief, especially when used with mild or moderately potent topical corticosteroid ointments. It is important to be very careful with dithranol, even in its short-contact form, because irritation may result. This may also apply to vitamin D analogues.

Case 8

An obese woman has psoriasis in her creases, for example, in her armpits, under her breasts or in her groin

It may help if she loses some weight to prevent the skin in the creases rubbing together. She should use moisturisers and mild topical corticosteroid products (such as hydrocortisone) or a moderately potent steroid such as clobetasone butyrate. The vitamin D analogue calcipotriol can be used with care, but it may sting, so she should use it only daily at first and build up to twice a day if it is tolerated.

CASE 9

A woman has severe nail psoriasis

There is no topical treatment that has consistently been shown to benefit patients with psoriasis of the nails. If she also has severe plaque psoriasis sufficient to warrant systemic treatment, then her nails may improve. She may also find that her nails improve spontaneously at any time.

Useful addresses

Psoriasis Association

7 Milton Street
Northampton NN2 7JG
Tel: 01604 711129
Fax: 01604 792894

This organisation provides information on different aspects of psoriasis, as well as promoting research. It produces a journal three times a year and organises an annual conference on psoriasis.

Psoriatic Arthropathy Alliance

PO Box 111
St Albans
Hertfordshire AL2 3JQ
Tel/fax: 01923 672837

This national registered charity raises awareness of psoriatic arthropathy. It provides information, produces a regular journal and puts people in touch with one another. You don't have to be a member if you wish to receive information or use the helpline.

British Association of Dermatologists

19 Fitzroy Square
London W1P 5HQ
Tel: 020 7383 0266
Fax: 020 7388 5263

This association represents dermatologists around the country. It provides members of the public with a list of dermatologists in their area, but does not recommend specific doctors. To consult a dermatologist, it is necessary to be referred by a GP.

Skin Care Campaign

An alliance of patient groups, companies and other organisations with a common interest in skin health. It is administered by the National Eczema Society.

Website: www.skincarecampaign.org

Index